GOLO DIET FOR SENIORS

Unlocking Vibrant Healthy Diet:
Seniors Golo Diet Hand Book

James Jackson

Table Of Content

Introduction

In a world marked by an ever-evolving parade of diets, each promising miraculous results, it's easy to feel lost amidst the cacophony of conflicting advice. But what if there were a dietary approach that transcended the transient trends and fads? What if there existed a nutritional journey uniquely tailored to the needs and aspirations of our most cherished generation, our seniors?

Welcome to a transformative journey, one that doesn't just promise health and well-being but embodies the very essence of ageing gracefully. In this age where wisdom and experience reign supreme, we present to you the "GOLO Diet for Seniors," a beacon of hope that shines brilliantly amid the challenges of growing older.

For our beloved seniors, each day marks another chapter in a life enriched with memories, wisdom, and invaluable contributions to society. But it also often brings with it the nuanced complexities of ageing—physical, mental, and emotional. The GOLO Diet for Seniors is not just another diet plan; it is a comprehensive testament to the power of scientific understanding, compassion, and an unwavering commitment to enhancing the quality of life during the golden years.

At its core, this journey is guided by one singular mission: to empower our seniors with the knowledge and tools necessary to reclaim vitality, reignite the spark of enthusiasm for life, and compose a compelling new chapter in their unique story of ageing with grace and gusto.

In this introduction, we invite you to embark on a voyage of rejuvenation and longevity, where the timeless wisdom of age is harmoniously intertwined with the cutting-edge science of nutrition. Together, we'll unravel the secrets behind the GOLO Diet's remarkable effectiveness in promoting metabolic health, hormonal balance, and overall well-being for seniors.

But first, let us explore the tapestry of ageing itself. What can one expect as the years roll on, and how can the GOLO Diet become your steadfast companion in this journey? What are the common health concerns that seniors face, and how can the power of nutrition be harnessed to navigate these challenges with poise and confidence?

Buckle up, dear reader, for the pages ahead are filled with insights, strategies, and success stories that will not only inform but inspire. It's time to embark on a voyage of transformation—one that celebrates the vibrancy of life, the wisdom of age, and the boundless potential of embracing the GOLO Diet for Seniors.

Are you ready to embark on a path that will not just transform your relationship with food but also your outlook on life? Join us as we dive deep into the heart of the GOLO Diet and embark on a journey that redefines ageing, one delicious and nutritious step at a time.

Chapter 1

Understanding Aging and Health

The Aging Process: What Seniors Should Expect

Ageing is a natural and inevitable part of life, a process that every individual experiences. While it can be a time of great fulfilment and contentment, it also brings various changes to both the body and mind. Understanding what seniors should expect during the ageing process is crucial for maintaining health and well-being in their later years.

Physical Changes:

1.Muscle Mass Reduction: With age, there is a gradual loss of muscle mass, a condition known as sarcopenia. Seniors may experience decreased strength and mobility.

2.Decreased Bone Density: Osteoporosis is a common concern for seniors, characterised by fragile bones that are more prone to fractures.

3.Slower Metabolism:Metabolism tends to slow down with age, making it easier to gain weight and more challenging to maintain a healthy weight.

4.Changes in Vision and Hearing:Seniors often experience changes in vision, such as presbyopia, cataracts, or macular degeneration. Hearing loss is also common.

5. Reduced Skin Elasticity: Skin becomes less elastic, leading to wrinkles and sagging.

Cognitive Changes

1. Slower Cognitive Processing: Seniors may notice that their cognitive processing speed is slower than in their younger years.

2. Memory Changes: Memory can be affected, with occasional forgetfulness being normal, but more severe memory issues could be signs of conditions like dementia.

Common Health Issues in Seniors

Several health concerns are prevalent among seniors. These include:

1. Cardiovascular Issues: Heart disease, hypertension, and stroke become more common as individuals age.

2.Diabetes: Type 2 diabetes risk increases with age, often due to changes in metabolism and lifestyle.

3. Arthritis: Conditions like osteoarthritis or rheumatoid arthritis can cause joint pain and decreased mobility.

4.Cancer: The risk of various cancers, such as breast, prostate, and lung cancer, increases with age.

5.Neurodegenerative Diseases: Conditions like Alzheimer's disease and Parkinson's disease are more likely to develop in older individuals.

6.Respiratory Conditions: Seniors are at greater risk of chronic obstructive pulmonary disease (COPD) and pneumonia.

7. Osteoporosis: Brittle bones can lead to fractures and increased injury risk.

8.<u>Vision and Hearing Problems</u>: Age-related vision and hearing issues, such as glaucoma, cataracts, or hearing loss, are common.

9.<u>Depression and Anxiety</u>:Mental health concerns can arise, often related to life changes, isolation, or medical conditions.

10.<u>Obesity</u>: Weight management can become challenging due to slower metabolism, muscle loss, and lifestyle changes.

Understanding these natural changes and potential health concerns is the first step in proactively addressing senior well-being. While ageing presents challenges, it also offers opportunities for personal growth, wisdom, and a fulfilling life. Seniors can maintain and even enhance their quality of life by staying informed, leading a healthy lifestyle, seeking regular medical check-ups, and connecting with a supportive community. Additionally, the GOLO Diet, as discussed earlier, provides a holistic approach to health that is tailored to the unique needs of seniors, addressing aspects of metabolic health, hormonal balance, and emotional well-being to support senior vitality.

Chapter 2

The Principles of the GOLO Diet

The GOLO Diet is not just another diet; it's a comprehensive wellness program meticulously designed to embrace the complexity of ageing. It beckons seniors to explore a holistic perspective on health, one that nurtures not only the physical body but also the spirit and mind guiding them through the intricate terrain of metabolic health, hormonal balance, and this is the unique aspects that set the GOLO Diet apart from conventional weight loss programs. It is a resource that will help you understand not just what to do but why you should do it, and how it can transform your life.

The ABCs of Metabolic Health

Metabolic health is a fundamental component of overall well-being, and understanding its ABCs is vital for seniors seeking to enhance their vitality and quality of life.

A: Aging and Metabolism: Aging naturally brings changes to the body's metabolism. As we age, our metabolic rate tends to slow down, and we may experience changes in the way our bodies process energy and nutrients.

The ABCs begin with "A" because it's essential for seniors to acknowledge and adapt to these age-related metabolic changes. The GOLO Diet recognizes that metabolic health is not a one-size-fits-all concept and should be tailored to individual needs.

B: Blood Sugar Control: Blood sugar, or glucose, plays a critical role in metabolic health. Seniors often face challenges in maintaining stable blood sugar levels, which can lead to a range of health issues.

Seniors should be aware of the impact of dietary choices on blood sugar and how to make better choices to keep it within a healthy range. The GOLO Diet places a strong focus on low-glycemic foods to support blood sugar control.

C: Comprehensive Approach: Metabolic health isn't just about what you eat; it's about the entire lifestyle you lead. Seniors need to take a comprehensive approach to manage their metabolic health successfully.

The GOLO Diet encourages a holistic perspective that combines proper nutrition, physical activity, stress management, and hormonal balance to support metabolic health. By addressing all these aspects, seniors can enhance their vitality and resilience.

Balancing Hormones for Senior Wellness

Hormonal balance is a pivotal aspect of senior wellness, and understanding how hormones affect health is crucial for making informed decisions regarding diet and lifestyle.

Understanding Hormonal Changes with Age

Ageing brings hormonal changes, including shifts in sex hormones, thyroid hormones, and insulin sensitivity. These changes can influence weight management, energy levels, and overall well-being. It's essential for seniors to be aware of these hormonal fluctuations, as they are part of the natural ageing process. The GOLO Diet acknowledges these changes and provides a framework to address them.

Impact of Hormonal Imbalances

Hormonal imbalances can lead to a host of health issues for seniors. For example, insulin resistance, a common issue as people age, can contribute to weight gain and increase the risk of diabetes. The GOLO Diet recognizes the far-reaching consequences of hormonal imbalances and focuses on strategies to mitigate these effects and promote overall wellness.

The GOLO Diet is designed to address hormonal imbalances by promoting nutrition that supports stable blood sugar levels, insulin sensitivity, and hormonal harmony. Embracing these principles focusing on the right foods, stress management, and physical activity, seniors can take meaningful steps toward a healthier, more fulfilling life.

Defining the GOLO Diet

The GOLO Diet is a wellness program specifically designed for seniors, although its principles can be applied to individuals of all ages. It takes a holistic approach to health, recognizing that well-being encompasses not only the physical aspect but also emotional and mental aspects. The central focus of the GOLO Diet is metabolic health and hormonal balance. It provides a framework that encourages seniors to make balanced and sustainable lifestyle changes, fostering overall vitality and longevity.

At its core, the GOLO Diet is about achieving metabolic balance and hormonal harmony. It acknowledges the complex interplay between nutrition, physical activity, stress management, and hormones in determining health outcomes. The GOLO Diet recognizes that seniors need tailored strategies to address their unique challenges, including age-related metabolic changes and hormonal fluctuations. It doesn't promote quick fixes or extreme dieting but encourages a long-term commitment to a healthier way of life.

The Holistic Philosophy of the GOLO Diet

The holistic philosophy of the GOLO Diet revolves around a few key principles:

1.Comprehensive Wellness: The GOLO Diet views wellness as a multifaceted concept that includes physical, emotional, and mental well-being. It emphasises that a healthy life is not just about the absence of disease but the presence of vitality and fulfilment.

2.Metabolic Health: Metabolism is at the heart of the GOLO Diet. It recognizes that how our bodies process energy and nutrients significantly impacts health. Thus, it encourages the consumption of foods that support stable blood sugar levels, weight management, and overall metabolic health.

3.Hormonal Balance: Hormones play a pivotal role in determining well-being. The GOLO Diet acknowledges the hormonal changes that come with ageing and provides strategies to address them. It particularly focuses on insulin sensitivity and blood sugar control to foster hormonal balance.

4.Lifestyle Integration: The GOLO Diet is not a quick fix; it's a sustainable lifestyle change. It encourages seniors to integrate wellness into their daily routines, ensuring that health-conscious choices become second nature.

5.Personalization: The GOLO Diet recognizes that every senior is unique. It encourages personalization, allowing individuals to tailor the program to their specific needs and preferences. This approach makes it accessible and practical for a wide range of seniors.

Unique Aspects of the GOLO Diet

The GOLO Diet stands out among wellness programs due to several unique aspects:

1.Balance Over Extremes: Unlike many fad diets that promote extreme calorie restrictions or the exclusion of entire food groups, the GOLO Diet emphasises balance. It promotes the consumption of real, whole foods in appropriate portions, making it more sustainable and enjoyable.

2.Blood Sugar Control: The GOLO Diet places a strong focus on controlling blood sugar levels through the consumption of low-glycemic foods. This emphasis on stable blood sugar not only supports metabolic health but also enhances overall well-being.

3.Emotional Wellness: The GOLO Diet recognizes the emotional aspect of health. It acknowledges the role of stress, emotional eating, and mental well-being in overall health. Stress management is an integral part of the program.

4.Senior-Centric Approach: While the principles of the GOLO Diet can benefit individuals of all ages, it is designed with seniors in mind. It takes into account the unique challenges faced by ageing individuals, providing tailored recommendations for this demographic.

The Importance of Holistic Wellness for Seniors

Holistic wellness is particularly important for seniors for several reasons:

1.Ageing Challenges: Aging often brings a host of health challenges, from metabolic changes to hormonal imbalances. Holistic wellness recognizes these challenges and offers solutions to mitigate their impact.

2.Quality of Life: Holistic wellness is not just about adding years to life but about adding life to years. It can enhance the quality of life for seniors by promoting vitality, energy, and emotional well-being.

3.Preventative Health: Holistic wellness focuses on prevention rather than reaction. It empowers seniors to proactively address health issues and reduce the risk of chronic diseases.

4.<u>Emotional Resilience:</u> Emotional and mental well-being is as crucial as physical health. Holistic wellness programs, like the GOLO Diet, acknowledge the importance of stress management and mental health support.

The GOLO Diet is more than a diet; it's a comprehensive wellness program designed to empower seniors to take control of their health. Its holistic philosophy recognizes the interplay of physical, emotional, and mental well-being, and it provides unique solutions to the challenges seniors face as they age. By embracing the GOLO Diet's principles, seniors can embark on a journey to a healthier, more fulfilling life in their golden years.

Chapter 3

THE GOLO DIET MEAL PLAN

GETTING STARTED

Practical tips for a successful GOLO Diet journey. The GOLO Diet is not just about what you eat but also how you integrate its principles into your daily life. These tips will help you make the most of this holistic approach to well-being:

1. Understand the Basics:
   Before you start, take the time to understand the core principles of the GOLO Diet. This includes metabolic health, hormonal balance, and emotional well-being. A strong foundation will guide your journey.

2. Set Clear Goals:
   Define your objectives. Whether it's weight loss, better blood sugar control, or increased vitality, having clear goals provides motivation and direction.

3. Plan Your Meals:
   Meal planning is a key aspect of success. Prepare balanced, GOLO Diet-friendly meals that incorporate lean protein, low-glycemic

carbohydrates, and vegetables. This helps control portions and maintain stable blood sugar levels.

4. Watch Portion Sizes:

   Be mindful of portion sizes to avoid overeating. Measuring your food, using smaller plates, and practising portion control will help you stay on track.

5. Stay Hydrated:

   Proper hydration is essential for overall well-being. Drinking enough water supports digestion, metabolism, and even helps control appetite.

6. Stock Your Kitchen Wisely:

   Fill your kitchen with GOLO Diet-approved foods. Having the right ingredients on hand makes it easier to prepare healthy meals.

7. Read Labels:

   When shopping, read food labels carefully. Look for products that are low in added sugars and high in fibre.

8. Incorporate Exercise:

   Physical activity is a vital part of the GOLO Diet. Aim for a mix of aerobic exercise and strength training. Consider low-impact activities that are gentle on the joints.

9. Manage Stress:

   Stress management is crucial. Incorporate relaxation techniques into your daily routine, such as deep breathing exercises, meditation, or yoga.

10. Stay Consistent:

Consistency is key to success. Make the GOLO Diet a lifestyle rather than a short-term endeavour. This will help you sustain results over time.

11. Monitor Your Progress:

Keep track of your journey. Regularly measure and assess your weight, blood sugar levels, and how you feel. Celebrate your successes, no matter how small.

12. Seek Support:

Consider joining a GOLO Diet community or support group. Sharing your experiences and challenges with like-minded individuals can provide encouragement and accountability.

13. Embrace Mindful Eating:

Pay attention to your food. Eating mindfully means savouring each bite and recognizing when you're full, preventing overeating.

14. Listen to Your Body:

Be attuned to your body's signals. If you're hungry, eat. If you're full, stop. Trust your body's cues.

15. Adapt and Personalise:

Remember that the GOLO Diet is flexible. Adjust it to your preferences, dietary restrictions, and specific needs. It should work for you, not the other way around.

16. Educate Yourself:

Continue to educate yourself about nutrition, exercise, and wellness. The more you know, the better equipped you are to make informed choices.

17. Be Patient:

Remember that lasting change takes time. Be patient with yourself and stay committed to the journey.

18. Consult a Professional:

If you have specific health concerns or questions, consider consulting a healthcare professional or a registered dietitian. They can offer tailored guidance and support.

19. Enjoy the Process:

Wellness is a journey, not a destination. Embrace the process, enjoy the changes you're making, and celebrate the improvements in your overall well-being.

20. Stay Positive:

Maintain a positive mindset. Believe in your ability to make lasting, positive changes, and your GOLO Diet journey will be all the more successful.

Establishing Achievable Health and Wellness Goals

Setting achievable health and wellness goals is a critical step in any wellness journey, including the GOLO Diet. Here's how to create goals that are both realistic and motivating:

1. Be Specific: Define your goals clearly. Instead of saying, "I want to lose weight," specify how much weight you want to lose and by when. Specific goals are easier to work towards.

2. Make Goals Measurable: Your goals should be quantifiable so that you can track your progress. Use concrete numbers, such as "lose 10 pounds" or "walk for 30 minutes a day."

3. Set Realistic Goals: Be honest with yourself about what you can realistically achieve. Unrealistic goals can lead to frustration. Consider your lifestyle, time constraints, and any health limitations.

4. Focus on Short-Term and Long-Term Goals: Create a mix of short-term and long-term goals. Short-term goals can provide quick wins and motivation, while long-term goals help you stay committed over time.

5. Prioritise Goals: Determine which goals are most important to you and focus your efforts on them.

Trying to achieve too many goals at once can be overwhelming.

6. Make Goals Time-Bound: Assign a timeframe to your goals. Having a deadline creates a sense of urgency and helps you stay on track.

7. Write Down Your Goals: Documenting your goals makes them feel more concrete and committed. Keep them somewhere visible, like on a vision board or in a journal.

Methods for Monitoring and Measuring Your Progress

Once you've set your goals, tracking your progress is essential to stay accountable and motivated. Here are practical methods for monitoring and measuring your progress on the GOLO Diet:

1. Keep a Food Journal: Record your daily meals, snacks, and water intake. This helps you see your eating patterns, identify potential challenges, and make adjustments as needed.

2. Weigh Yourself Regularly: Weighing yourself once a week can provide insights into your weight loss progress. However, remember that weight is just one measure of health. Don't get discouraged by occasional fluctuations.

3. Take Body Measurements: In addition to weight, track your body measurements, such as waist,

hips, and chest. These measurements can reveal changes in body composition, even when the scale doesn't move.

4. Blood Sugar Monitoring: If you have diabetes or are working on blood sugar control, regularly check your blood glucose levels. This provides immediate feedback on the impact of your dietary choices.

5. Fitness Tracking: Use fitness apps or wearables to track your physical activity. This can help you monitor your exercise frequency, duration, and intensity.

6. Keep a Mood Journal: Track your emotional well-being. Note how you're feeling, stress levels, and any emotional triggers related to eating. This can help you manage emotional eating.

7. Photos: Take "before" and progress photos to visually assess changes in your body. Sometimes, visual evidence of your progress can be motivating.

8. Self-Reflection: Regularly take some time to reflect on your wellness journey. Assess how you're feeling, what's working, and what needs adjustment.

9. Goal Review: Periodically review your goals to see if they're still relevant and achievable. Adjust them as necessary to stay aligned with your evolving needs.

10. Celebrate Milestones: Recognize and celebrate your achievements, even small ones. Rewards and acknowledgment can keep you motivated.

11. Consult a Healthcare Professional: For specific health concerns, regular check-ups and consultations with healthcare professionals can provide valuable insights into your progress.

Monitoring and measuring your progress not only helps you stay on track but also empowers you with the knowledge needed to make informed decisions on your GOLO Diet journey. These methods allow you to assess what's working, identify areas for improvement, and maintain a proactive approach to your health and well-being.

Here's a simple one-week meal plan for the GOLO Diet to help you get started.
These meal ideas include recipes for breakfast, lunch, and dinner, as well as some additional recipe ideas for variety. We'll also discuss smart snacking and hydration to help you stay on track.

Day 1
Breakfast:
- Scrambled eggs with spinach and tomatoes
- Whole-grain toast
Lunch:

- Grilled chicken salad with mixed greens, cucumbers, and vinaigrette dressing

Dinner:
- Baked salmon with lemon and dill
- Quinoa
- Steamed broccoli

Day 2
Breakfast:
- Greek yoghourt with berries and honey
Lunch:
- Lentil soup
- Mixed greens salad with olive oil and balsamic vinegar
Dinner:
- Grilled lean pork loin
- Roasted sweet potatoes
- Steamed asparagus

Day 3
Breakfast:
- Oatmeal with sliced banana and a sprinkle of almonds
Lunch:
- Tuna salad (canned tuna, mixed with light mayo, and chopped veggies)
- Whole-grain crackers
Dinner:
- Stir-fried tofu with mixed vegetables and a low-sodium soy sauce

- Brown rice

Day 4

Breakfast:

- Whole-grain pancakes with fresh fruit

Lunch:

- Quinoa salad with chickpeas, cucumbers, and a lemon-tahini dressing

Dinner:

- Grilled shrimp with garlic and herbs
- Couscous
- Steamed green beans

Day 5:

Breakfast:

- Veggie omelette with mushrooms, bell peppers, and onions

Lunch:

- Turkey and avocado wrap in a whole-grain tortilla

Dinner:

- Baked chicken breast with rosemary
- Mashed cauliflower
- Roasted Brussels sprouts

Day 6

Breakfast:

- Cottage cheese with sliced peaches

Lunch:

- Spinach and feta stuffed chicken breast

- Quinoa salad
Dinner:
- Grilled sirloin steak with a side of sautéed kale
- Baked sweet potato

Day 7
Breakfast:
- Smoothie with spinach, banana, and a scoop of protein powder
Lunch:
- Caprese salad with fresh mozzarella, tomatoes, and basil
Dinner:
- Baked cod with a lemon herb marinade
- Wild rice
- Steamed carrots

Additional Recipe Ideas for Variety:
1. Veggie Stir-Fry: Sauté a mix of colourful vegetables with tofu or lean protein and a low-sodium stir-fry sauce.
2. Mediterranean Bowl: Create a bowl with hummus, falafel, tabbouleh, and a variety of fresh veggies.
3. Quinoa and Black Bean Salad: Mix cooked quinoa with black beans, corn, red pepper, and a lime-cilantro dressing.

4. Zucchini Noodles with Pesto: Use a spiralizer to create zucchini noodles and toss them with homemade or store-bought pesto.
5. Salmon with Mango Salsa: Top grilled salmon with a fresh mango salsa for a burst of flavour.

Smart Snacking

- Opt for whole, unprocessed snacks like fresh fruit, raw nuts, or Greek yoghurt.
- Prepare small portions of snack-size veggies and hummus.
- Consider homemade energy balls made with oats, nuts, and dried fruit.

Hydration Guide

- Aim to drink at least 8 glasses (64 ounces) of water daily.
- Herbal teas and infused water with slices of fruit or cucumber are great alternatives.
- Limit sugary beverages and soda; opt for water or unsweetened herbal teas instead.

Remember to adapt the meal plan and recipes to your specific preferences and dietary needs. The key to success on the GOLO Diet is to enjoy a variety of whole, unprocessed foods that support metabolic health and overall well-being while staying hydrated and making smart snacking choices.

Chapter 4

Exercise And Movement For Seniors

Importance of Physical Activity for Seniors

Staying physically active is crucial for seniors' health and well-being. Here are some key reasons why maintaining an active lifestyle is so important for older individuals:

1. Maintains Mobility and Independence: Regular physical activity helps preserve muscle strength and joint flexibility, enabling seniors to perform daily activities independently.

2. Enhances Cardiovascular Health: Exercise improves heart health by reducing the risk of heart disease, high blood pressure, and stroke. It also promotes better circulation.

3. Weight Management: Staying active helps manage body weight, reducing the risk of obesity and related health issues, such as diabetes and joint problems.

4. Enhances Bone Health: Weight-bearing exercises like walking, dancing, and strength training can help maintain bone density and reduce the risk of osteoporosis and fractures.

5. Cognitive Benefits: Physical activity has been linked to improved cognitive function and a

reduced risk of age-related cognitive decline, including conditions like dementia.

6. Stress Reduction: Exercise is an excellent stress reliever, helping seniors manage emotional well-being and mental health.

7. Social Engagement: Many physical activities, like group fitness classes or walking clubs, provide opportunities for social interaction, reducing feelings of isolation.

8. Better Sleep: Regular exercise can improve sleep quality, which is important for overall health and well-being.

Choosing Appropriate Exercises for Seniors

Selecting exercises that are suitable for one's fitness level and health is crucial to ensure safety and effectiveness. Here are some considerations when choosing exercises:

1. Consult a Healthcare Professional: Before beginning any exercise program, consult with a healthcare provider to assess your health status and receive personalised recommendations.

2. Start Slowly: If you're new to exercise or haven't been active for a while, start with low-intensity activities like walking. Gradually increase intensity and duration over time.

3. Balance Activities: A well-rounded fitness routine includes aerobic exercises (e.g., walking, swimming), strength training (with light weights

or resistance bands), and flexibility exercises (like yoga or stretching).

4. Adapt for Health Conditions: If you have specific health concerns or conditions, such as arthritis, consult a physical therapist or fitness professional to adapt exercises accordingly.

5. Listen to Your Body: Pay attention to how your body responds to exercise. If you experience pain or discomfort, modify or discontinue the activity and seek advice from a healthcare professional.

Practical Tips for Incorporating More Movement into Daily Life

1. Take Short Walks: Aim to take short walks throughout the day, even if it's just around your home or office. Short, frequent walks can add up.

2. Use Household Chores: Engage in activities like gardening, cleaning, or cooking that require movement. These are effective ways to stay active and accomplish daily tasks.

3. Join a Fitness Class: Participating in senior-specific fitness classes can provide structure and social interaction. Many communities offer such classes.

4. Use a Pedometer: Tracking your steps with a pedometer can be motivating. Set a daily step goal and gradually increase it.

5. Take the Stairs: Whenever possible, choose stairs over elevators or escalators. It's an easy way to

incorporate more movement into your daily routine.

6. Dance: Put on your favourite music and dance in the living room. Dancing is an enjoyable and pleasant way to stay active.

7. Stay Consistent: Create a routine that includes physical activity and make it a part of your daily life. Consistency is key to reaping the benefits of exercise.

8. Find a Workout Buddy: Exercising with a friend or family member can provide motivation and make it more enjoyable.

Incorporating movement into your daily life doesn't have to be complicated or time-consuming. It's about finding activities you enjoy, staying consistent, and adapting to your fitness level and health needs. Physical activity is a lifelong investment in your health, and it's never too late to start or continue an active lifestyle as a senior.

Managing Stress And Sleep

Stress Reduction Techniques for Seniors

Managing stress is essential for seniors as it is often linked to various health issues, including heart disease, high blood pressure, and mental health concerns. Here are some stress reduction techniques and strategies for seniors:

1. Mindfulness Meditation: Practising mindfulness helps seniors become more aware of the present moment, reducing anxiety and stress. Techniques like deep breathing, body scans, and meditation can be highly beneficial.

2. Yoga: Yoga combines physical postures, breathing exercises, and meditation to reduce stress and improve flexibility. There are modified yoga classes specifically designed for seniors.

3. Exercise: Regular physical activity releases endorphins, which are natural mood lifters. Activities like walking, swimming, or tai chi can also be both physically and mentally beneficial.

4. Social Interaction: Engaging with friends and loved ones can alleviate feelings of loneliness and isolation, reducing stress. Join clubs or social groups to foster connections.

5. Journaling: Keeping a journal allows seniors to express their thoughts and feelings, which can be a cathartic way to manage stress and gain perspective.

6. Cognitive Behavioral Therapy (CBT): CBT can help seniors reframe negative thought patterns and learn effective coping strategies for stress.

7. Music and Art Therapy: Engaging in creative activities like painting, drawing, or playing a

musical instrument can be relaxing and therapeutic.

8. Nature Walks: Spending time in nature, whether it's a park or a garden, has a calming effect and can reduce stress.

Improving Sleep Quality

Quality sleep is crucial for overall health, and seniors often struggle with sleep-related issues. Here are tips to enhance sleep quality:

1. Establish a Routine: Go to bed and wake up at the same time every day, even on weekends, to regulate your body's internal clock.

2. Create a Relaxing Bedtime Routine: Engage in calming activities before bed, such as reading, taking a warm bath, or practising relaxation techniques.

3. Optimise Your Sleep Environment: Ensure your bedroom is dark, quiet, and at a comfortable temperature. Invest in a comfortable mattress and pillows.

4. Limit Screen Time: Avoid screens (phones, tablets, TVs) at least an hour before bedtime as the blue light can disrupt sleep patterns.

5. Watch Your Diet: Avoid heavy meals and caffeine close to bedtime. However, a light snack,

like a small piece of fruit, can help prevent hunger from keeping you awake.

6. Exercise Regularly: Engaging in physical activity during the day can help you fall asleep faster and enjoy deeper sleep. Just avoid vigorous exercise close to bedtime.

7. Manage Stress: Practice stress reduction techniques (as mentioned earlier) to alleviate anxiety and relax the mind before sleep.

8. Limit Naps: While short naps can be refreshing, long or frequent naps during the day can interfere with nighttime sleep.

Enhancing Mental and Emotional Health

1. Stay Mentally Active: Engage in activities that challenge your mind, such as puzzles, reading, or learning new skills. Lifelong learning is beneficial for mental health.

2. Seek Professional Help: If you're struggling with mental health concerns, don't hesitate to consult a mental health professional. Therapy and counselling can provide valuable support.

3. Stay Socially Active: Maintaining social connections is essential for emotional health. Regularly interact with friends and family, and consider joining clubs or groups of interest.

4. Volunteer: Giving back to the community through volunteering can provide a sense of purpose and satisfaction, enhancing emotional well-being.
5. Practice Gratitude: Regularly reflect on things you're grateful for. This simple practice can boost mood and well-being.
6. Maintain a Positive Outlook: Focus on the positives in life and practice self-compassion. Avoid dwelling on negative thoughts.
7. Stay Active: Physical activity not only benefits physical health but also has a profound impact on mental and emotional well-being. It releases endorphins, which are natural mood boosters.

By incorporating these stress reduction techniques, sleep improvement strategies, and practices to enhance mental and emotional health into your daily routine, you can enjoy a happier, healthier, and more fulfilling senior lifestyle.

Chapter 5

Medication Management Dealing With Common Age Related Challenge

Managing Medications and Interactions with the GOLO Diet

Managing medications alongside the GOLO Diet is crucial for seniors, especially when dealing with age-related health concerns. Here's some guidance:

1. Consult Your Healthcare Provider: Before starting any new diet plan, including the GOLO Diet, it's essential to discuss it with your healthcare provider. They can evaluate your current medications and adjust them if necessary.

2. Medication Timing: Some medications may need to be taken with food, while others should be taken on an empty stomach. Understand the requirements of your specific medications and coordinate them with your meal plan.

3. Monitor Blood Sugar Levels:If you're on medications for diabetes, closely monitor your blood sugar levels as you make dietary changes. You may need adjustments to your medication to prevent hypoglycemia (low blood sugar).

4. Be Aware of Potential Interactions: Some medications may interact with certain foods or supplements. Talk to your healthcare provider

about any potential interactions with the foods or supplements recommended on the GOLO Diet.

5. Stay Hydrated: Medications can sometimes lead to dehydration. Ensure you're staying well-hydrated by drinking plenty of water throughout the day.

6. Adhere to Medication Schedules: Take your medications as prescribed, and use tools like pill organisers to help you stay organised and avoid missing doses.

Strategies for Addressing Age-Related Challenges

As seniors face age-related issues, it's important to adopt strategies that enhance overall well-being:

1. Regular Health Check-Ups: Schedule regular check-ups with your healthcare provider to monitor age-related conditions such as heart disease, osteoporosis, and cancer.

2. Nutrition for Bone Health: Consume foods rich in calcium and vitamin D to support bone health. Supplements may be necessary if dietary intake is insufficient.

3. Exercise Safely: Engage in exercise that is appropriate for your fitness level, considering any existing health conditions. Low-impact exercises like swimming and tai chi are gentle on the joints.

4. Mental Stimulation: Keep your mind active through puzzles, reading, and lifelong learning. This can help prevent cognitive decline.

5. Prevent Falls: Make your living space safe by removing tripping hazards, installing handrails, and using assistive devices if needed.

6. Manage Chronic Conditions: If you have chronic conditions like diabetes or high blood pressure, adhere to your treatment plan and maintain regular check-ups.

7. Stay Socially Active: Loneliness and isolation can be detrimental to mental and emotional health. Stay socially active through clubs, groups, and community activities.

8. Adapt to Lifestyle Changes: As your needs change with age, be open to adjusting your lifestyle. This might include downsizing your home, transitioning to a retirement community, or seeking home health assistance if necessary.

9. Address Emotional Well-Being: Mental health is as important as physical health. Seek support from mental health professionals or counsellors if you're experiencing emotional challenges.

10. Stay Informed: Stay informed about age-related conditions and lifestyle modifications that can support your health. Education is a powerful tool for self-advocacy.

Addressing age-related challenges requires a combination of medical guidance, self-care, and adaptability. The GOLO Diet, with its focus on metabolic health, can complement these strategies by providing a foundation for better nutrition and overall wellness, supporting seniors in their quest for a healthy and fulfilling life.

Conclusion

In the journey of exploring the GOLO Diet for seniors, you've embarked on a path towards enhanced well-being, embracing the principles of metabolic health, hormonal balance, and emotional well-being. This holistic approach is designed to empower you to take control of your health and vitality, regardless of your age.

As you conclude this book, remember that your wellness journey is ongoing. The wisdom you've gained here is just the beginning. To continue your success and further your understanding of the GOLO Diet and its applications, consider these additional resources and tools:

1. GOLO Diet Official Website: The official GOLO Diet website offers a wealth of information, including meal plans, success stories, and access to tools and community support.

2. Books and Cookbooks: Explore additional books and cookbooks dedicated to the GOLO Diet to expand your knowledge and discover new recipes.

3. Online Communities: Join online forums, social media groups, or communities dedicated to the GOLO Diet. Here, you can connect with others, share experiences, and gain motivation.

4. Mobile Apps: There are various mobile apps available to help you track your meals, physical activity, and progress. They can be convenient tools for staying on track.

5. Registered Dietitian Consultation: If you have specific dietary concerns or health conditions, consider

consulting with a registered dietitian who can provide personalised guidance.

6. Fitness Classes and Programs: Explore local fitness classes, wellness programs, or personal trainers who can help you design a fitness plan tailored to your needs.

7. Meditation and Mindfulness Apps: Discover apps and resources for meditation and mindfulness to support emotional well-being and stress management.

8. Sleep Tracking Devices: Invest in sleep tracking devices or apps that can provide insights into your sleep patterns and help you optimise your sleep quality.

9. Library and Academic Resources: Continue your education by visiting your local library or exploring academic resources on topics related to nutrition, health, and wellness.

10. Healthcare Professionals: Don't hesitate to consult your healthcare provider or other specialists as needed to address specific health concerns and receive tailored guidance.

Your journey towards well-being is a lifelong adventure, and the knowledge and tools you've acquired will serve as a foundation for lasting change. Remember that you have the power to shape your health and vitality. As you continue your path, stay inspired, stay determined, and embrace each day as an opportunity to be the healthiest, happiest version of yourself. Your future is bright, and your potential is limitless. Keep going, keep growing, and keep thriving on the GOLO Diet.

Golo Diet For Seniors

Made in the USA
Las Vegas, NV
04 September 2024

94790894R10036